Intermittent Fasting for Women Over 50

The Essential Guide to Lose Weight Fast, Detox Your Body, Reset and Speed Up Your Metabolism

Angela Boston

© **Copyright 2021 by Angela Boston**

All rights reserved

This document is geared towards providing exact and reliable information in regards to the topic and issue covered. The publication is sold with the idea that the publisher is not required to render accounting, officially permitted, or otherwise, qualified services. If advice is necessary, legal or professional, a practiced individual in the profession should be ordered.

- From a Declaration of Principles which was accepted and approved equally by a Committee of the American Bar Association and a Committee of Publishers and Associations.

In no way is it legal to reproduce, duplicate, or transmit any part of this document in either electronic means or in printed format. Recording of this publication is strictly prohibited and any storage of this document is not allowed unless with written permission from the publisher. All rights reserved.

The information provided herein is stated to be truthful and consistent, in that any liability, in terms of inattention or otherwise, by any usage or abuse of any policies, processes, or directions contained within is the solitary and utter responsibility of the recipient reader. Under no circumstances will any legal responsibility or blame be held against the publisher for any reparation, damages, or monetary loss due to the information herein, either directly or indirectly.

Respective authors own all copyrights not held by the publisher.

The information herein is offered for informational purposes solely, and is universal as so. The presentation of the information is without contract or any type of guarantee assurance.

The trademarks that are used are without any consent, and the publication of the trademark is without permission or backing by the trademark owner. All trademarks and brands within this book are for clarifying purposes only and are the owned by the owners themselves, not affiliated with this document.

Contents

INTRODUCTION 9

CHAPTER 1: INTERMITTENT FASTING 11

1.1 WHY YOU NEED TO CONSIDER INTERMITTENT FASTING AS YOUR BEST CHOICE IF YOU ARE OVER 50. 12
1.2 WHY INTERMITTENT FASTING IS A BETTER CHOICE OVER ANY STRICT DIET. 14
1.3 AUTOPHAGY AND ITS RELATIONSHIP WITH INTERMITTENT FASTING. 17
1.4 INTERMITTENT FASTING TYPES 21
1.5 TIPS AND TRICKS TO MAKE THE MOST OUT OF INTERMITTENT FASTING. 34
1.6 COMMON MISTAKES PEOPLE DO WHEN APPROACHING INTERMITTENT FASTING. 46

CHAPTER 2: HOW TO BEGIN WITH INTERMITTENT FASTING 52

2.1 DETERMINE YOUR PERSONAL OBJECTIVES. 53
2.2 SELECT A METHOD. 54
2.3 DETERMINE YOUR CALORIE REQUIREMENTS 57
2.4 CREATE A MEAL PLAN. 57
2.5 KEEP TRACK OF YOUR CALORIES. 58
2.6 EXERCISE-RELATED EFFECTS 58

CHAPTER 3: INTERMITTENT FASTING HEALTH BENEFITS FOR WOMEN OVER 50 59

3.1 CARDIOVASCULAR HEALTH 59
3.2 DIABETES 60
3.3 LOSS OF WEIGHT 61
3.4 IT MIGHT ASSIST YOU IN EATING LESS 62

3.5 Fat-burning and Noradrenaline 63
3.6 Defend Against Oxidative Stress 63
3.7 Increases Life Expectancy 63
3.8 Other Health Advantages 63

CHAPTER 4: HOW INTERMITTENT FASTING WORKS FOR WOMEN OVER 50 65

4.1 Pros and Cons of Intermittent Fasting for Women Over 50 (And Why It Can Get Tricky) 67
4.2 The Best Intermittent Fasting Techniques For Women Over 50 69
4.3 When Should Intermittent Fasting Be Avoided? 70
4.4 Side Effects and Safety 71
4.5 Tips on Getting Started 72

CHAPTER 5: KINDS OF INTERMITTENT FASTING THAT WORK BEST FOR WOMEN 74

CHAPTER 6: FOODS WOMEN OVER 50 EAT SHOULD EAT IN INTERMITTENT FASTING 77

6.1 Water 79
6.2 Avocado 79
6.3 Seafood and fish 80
6.4 Cruciferous vegetables 81
6.5 Potatoes 81
6.6 Legumes and beans 81
6.7 Probiotics 82
6.8 Berry 82
6.9 Eggs 83
6.10 Nuts and seeds 83
6.11 Consume whole grains 84

CHAPTER 7: FOODS WOMEN OVER 50 SHOULD AVOID 85

7.1 SUGAR 85
7.2 AERATED BEVERAGES 85
7.3 PRODUCTS DERIVED FROM MILK 85
7.4 MEAT 86
7.5 ALCOHOL 86
7.6 CARBOHYDRATES 86
7.7 FOODS THAT HAVE BEEN FRIED 87
7.8 SALT IN EXCESS 87

CHAPTER 8: WEEKLY MEAL PLAN FOR WOMEN OVER 50 88

DAY 1 89
DAY 2 89
DAY 3 90
DAY 4 90
DAY 5 90
DAY 6 91
DAY 7 91

CHAPTER 9: FREQUENTLY ASKED QUESTIONS 92

CONCLUSION 97

Introduction

You may have heard the term "Intermittent Fasting" from time to time. Despite how frightening the name may appear, this strategy is simple to implement. It was also named the most popular weight-loss approach in 2019. If you've tried fasting before, you'll find that intermittent fasting isn't difficult to follow. It's also not necessary to be familiar with the notion of fasting to practice intermittent fasting. Intermittent fasting has gained popularity around the world, and many people practice it regularly. This has much more advantages than you may realize. And, if you're unfamiliar with Intermittent Fasting, or IF for short, it won't make you starve yourself. It also doesn't permit you to eat a lot of unhealthy food while you aren't fasting. Rather than eating meals & snacks throughout the day, people eat within a set period.

The majority of people adhere to an IF regimen that requires individuals to fast from 12 - 16 hours per day. They consume regular meals and snacks the majority of the time. Since most people are sleeping for roughly eight hours during their fasting hours, sticking to this eating window isn't as difficult as it sounds. You're also recommended to drink zero-calorie beverages, including water, tea, & coffee. Fast Bars can also be eaten in between meals to keep the fast going.

Women over 50 may benefit from intermittent fasting to lose weight and reduce their risk of acquiring age-related disorders.

Achy joints, Lower metabolism, diminished muscle mass, & even sleep troubles all make it more difficult to lose weight beyond 50. Simultaneously, decreasing fat, particularly harmful belly fat, can significantly lower your chance of serious health problems, including diabetes, heart attacks, & cancer.

Of fact, as you get older, your chances of contracting a variety of ailments rise. When it comes to losing weight and reducing the risk of acquiring age-related disorders, intermittently fast for women over 50 may be a real fountain of youth in some circumstances.

Intermittent fasting is one of the most popular health & fitness trends in the world right now.

People are using it to lose weight, enhance their health, and simplify their lives.

Many studies have shown that it could have a significant impact on your body & brain and that it may even increase longevity.

This is the ultimate guide to intermittent fasting for women over the age of 50.

Chapter 1: Intermittent Fasting

Intermittent fasting is a way of eating, not a diet. It's a method of planning your meals, and you'll get the most bang for your buck. Intermittent fasting does not alter you're eating habits; rather, it alters the timing of your meals.

Most importantly, it's a wonderful technique and gets slim without going on either a fad diet or severely restricting your calorie intake. When you first start intermittent fasting, you'll want to maintain your calorie intake constant. (Most people have larger meals in a shorter period.) Intermittent fasting is also an effective strategy to maintain muscle mass while losing weight.

The primary motivation for people to try intermittent fasting would be to lose some weight. In a moment, we'll speak about just how intermittent fasting helps you lose weight.

Most significantly, because it needs very little behavior change, intermittent fasting has been one of the simplest treatments we have for losing weight while maintaining a healthy weight. This is a positive thing since it suggests intermittent fasting fits into the category of "easy enough to perform, but meaningful enough to make a difference."

1.1 Why You Need to Consider Intermittent Fasting as Your Best Choice if You Are Over 50.

Lower metabolism, reduced muscle mass, achy joints, and even sleep problems all make it more difficult to lose weight after 50. At the same time, losing weight, including harmful belly fat, will significantly lower the risk of major health problems, including diabetes, heart attacks, and cancer. Of course, when you get older, the chances of contracting a variety of diseases rise. When it comes to weight reduction and that the risk of developing age-related ailments, intermittent fasting for women over 50 can be a virtual fountain of youth in certain situations. Some people claim that IF has helped them lose weight mainly because the short eating window forces them to eat fewer calories. For example, instead of three meals and two snacks, they can only have time for two meals and one snack. They become more conscious about the foods they eat and prefer to avoid unhealthy fats, processed carbohydrates, and empty calories. Of course, you have the freedom to choose any nutritious foods you choose. While certain people use intermittent fasting to limit their daily calorie consumption, some use it in conjunction with a keto, vegan, or any other diet.

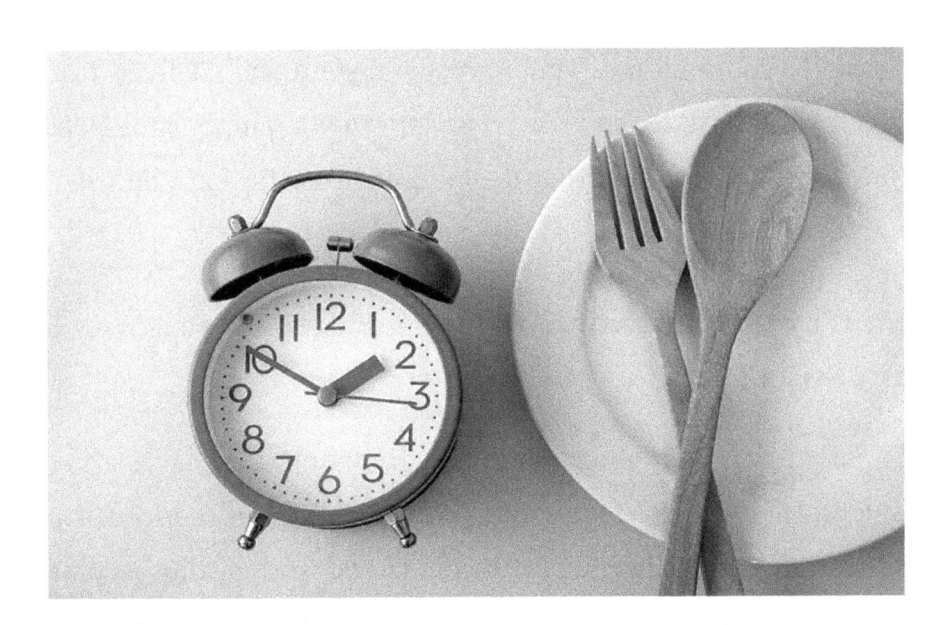

Benefits of Intermittent Fasting for Women Might Go Beyond Calorie Limitation

Although some nutritionists claim that IF only succeeds that in allows people to consume less, others dispute. They assume that with the same number of calories and other nutrients, intermittent fasting produces greater effects than traditional meal plans. Studies have also proposed that fasting for many hours a day accomplishes more than mere calorie restriction.

These are some of the metabolic modifications that IF induces, which can further explain the synergistic effects:

- Insulin: Lower insulin levels during the fasting period can aid fat burning.
- HGH: HGH levels increase as insulin levels fall, promoting fat burning and muscle development.

- Noradrenaline: The nervous system will deliver this chemical to cells in reaction to an empty stomach, informing them that they must release fat for food.

1.2 Why Intermittent Fasting is a Better Choice Over any Strict Diet.

There are numerous advantages to maintaining a healthy weight. Diabetes risk is lowered, joint discomfort is reduced, the danger of some cancers is lowered, and the cardiovascular system is overall healthier. Some diets, particularly a Mediterranean diet, appear to be particularly well suited to providing these benefits, albeit, as with other diets, this is contingent on people's ability to stick to them and prevent overeating. According to new research, another popular diet may provide even more health benefits. At least, that's the premise of some researchers studying intermittent fasting, a method of eating and not eating.

Intermittent fasting (IF) is based on decades of research indicating that feeding rats every other day keeps them thin and helps them acquire fewer aging-related illnesses and live 30 - 40 percent longer. Gerontologist Rafael del Cabo of said National Institute on Ageing and neurologist Mark Mattson at Johns Hopkins presented various data in animals and a smaller number in humans in a review article published in British Medical Journal in 2019. Suppose it is a real fountain of youth in rats and, to some extent in monkeys, lowering body mass, blood pressure, and cholesterol levels, enhancing lipid levels, reducing oxidative stress, maintaining brain function, and increasing endurance and coordination. Various kinds of IF have been found in human trials to be successful ways to exercise, regulate blood sugar, & lower blood pressure. There are suggestions that the more rigorous forms—those involving longer or tighter fasts—offer more benefits. "However, to be honest, many of the benefits we detect in animals don't translate to human beings," adds Krista Varady, a nutrition expert only at the University of Illinois. "This isn't a miracle diet."

Alternate-day fasting, in which individuals differ among feast days (usually eating maybe a little more) and fast days (eating only one small meal of about 500 calories); the 5:2 plan, in which people normally eat 5 days a week but only one small meal the other two days; as well as time-restricted eating, in which daily eateries is confined to an eight-hour window (or, in some, six 10 hours).

Many of the benefits of intermittent fasting are attributed to a process known as metabolic switching, in which the system depletes its store of glucose (a store polymer of sugar) and begins burning ketone (a fuel made from the fat by the liver). Growth factors, immunological signals, and other substances are all affected by this switch. But, as Mattson points out, ketones aren't the whole issue. "These episodes of skipping breakfast activate genes and signaling pathways that render neurons extra resilient," he claims, citing animal studies as evidence. "It triggers a process known as autophagy, in which cells are in a stress-resistance & recycling mode, removing damaged proteins." According to Mattson, fasting and eating cycles are similar to exercise and rest: "Your muscles don't become bigger during activity; they become bigger after recovery."

There is strong evidence that IF aids weight loss. Two trials, each including around 100 older women, evaluated the 5:2 diet to a diet that reduced daily calories by 25%; both discovered that the following diets resulted in the same weight - loss over 3 to 6 months. On the other hand, the intermittent fasters had better blood sugar management and lost more body fat. In addition, Varady's team found that alternate-day fasting enhanced the body's sensitivity to insulin by and over twice more than a standard calorie-cutting diet in a 2019 study with 43 overweight persons.

According to Courtney Peterson, an assistant registered dietitian belongs from the University of Alabama at Birmingham, IF may help lower blood pressure. Peterson's lab found that confining meals to a 6-hour window that concluded at 3 p.m. improved insulin sensitivity & blood pressure without weight loss in small yet rigorous research with prediabetes males IF is also being tested in dozens of clinical trials to see if it can prevent cancer growth and relieve symptoms of sclerosis, stroke, Ulcerative colitis, and other disorders.

1.3 Autophagy and its Relationship with Intermittent Fasting.

1.3.1 What exactly is autophagy?

According to Priya Khorana, Ph.D., in proper nutrition at Columbia University, autophagy is the body's mechanism of clearing out damaged cells to create younger, healthier cells.

The words "autophagy" and "auto" signify "self" and "eat," respectively. As a result, autophagy means "self-eating."

It's also known as "self-devouring." While it may sound like someone you'd rather not happen in your body, it's really good for your general health.

According to deck cardiologist Dr. Luiza Petre, autophagy is an adaptive ego-system by which the body may remove damaged cells and recycle portions of them toward coordination problems and cleaning.

The goal of autophagy, according to Petre, is to eliminate garbage and self-regulate back towards optimal smooth performance.

"It's like pressing a reset button on your body because it recycles and cleans at the same time. Additionally, it aids survival and adaptation in response to numerous stressors and poisons accumulating in our cells," she says.

1.3.2 What are the benefits of autophagy?

The major benefits of autophagy appear to be anti-aging concepts. It's best recognized, according to Petre, as the body's mechanism of turning back the clock and producing younger cells.

According to Khorana, whenever our cells are distressed, autophagy increases to protect us; this helps extend our lives.

According to registered dietitian Scotty Keatley, RD, CDN, through breaking cellular material & reusing it for vital processes.

"Of course, this requires energy and cannot be sustained indefinitely," he says, "but it allows us more time to obtain nourishment."

Autophagy has several advantages only at the cellular level, according to Petre:

eliminating harmful proteins from cells, which are linked to neurological illnesses like Parkinson's and Alzheimer's use leftover proteins supplying energy PPP & building blocks to cells that can still be repaired It promotes the regeneration of healthy cells on a greater scale Autophagy is also attracting a lot of support because of its potential role in cancer prevention and treatment.

"As we age, autophagy diminishes, so cells which no longer work and may cause harm are free to expand, which is cancer cells' MO," explains Keatley.

While all malignancies begin with faulty cells, according to Petre, the body should recognize and eliminate those cells frequently through autophagic processes. As a result, several researchers are investigating whether autophagy can minimize the chances of cancer.

While there is no scientific proof to support this, Petre claims that some studies Trusted Source shows that autophagy can destroy many malignant cells.

She continues, "It's how the body enforces the cancer villains." "Recognizing & destroying what went wrong, as well as starting the healing mechanism, helps to reduce cancer risk."

According to the researchers, fresh research will lead to new insights that will enable scientists to address autophagy as a cancer therapy.

1.3.3. Intermittent Fasting and Autophagy

Autophagy is a word that simply implies "self-eating." Intermittent fasting and ketogenic diets are believed to cause autophagy, which makes sense.

The most powerful way to trigger autophagy is by fasting.

Ketosis, a high-fat, low-carbohydrate diet, has the same advantages of fasting without the fasting, acting as a shortcut to cause the same beneficial metabolic changes. It allows the body a break by not overloading it with an external load, allowing it to concentrate on its own wellbeing and repair."

You receive about 75 percent of the recommended daily calories from fat on the keto diet, and 5 to 10% of your calories from carbohydrates. Your body's metabolic processes shift as a result of the change in calorie sources. It would begin to use fat as a source of energy rather than glucose obtained from carbohydrates.

As a consequence of this limitation, the body will continue to develop ketone bodies, which have various defensive properties. Studies show that ketosis may cause starvation-induced autophagy, which has neuroprotective properties

. Low glucose levels are related to low insulin and elevated glucagon levels in both diets. And it is the glucagon degree that triggers autophagy.

When the body is low on sugar due to fasting or ketosis, it causes beneficial stress, which activates the survival restoring mode.

Exercise is one non-diet factor that can play a role in autophagy induction. Physical exercise may induce autophagy in organs involved in metabolic regulation processes.

Muscles, pancreas, liver, and adipose tissue can be included in this.

1.4 Intermittent Fasting Types

Intermittent fasting has been a common health trend in recent years. It is said to help people lose weight, boost their metabolic health, and maybe even live longer. This eating trend may be approached in a variety of ways. Every method can be effective but determining which one works best for you is a personal decision.

1. 16:8

Sort 16:8 intermittent fasting is a type of time-restricted fasting. It requires eating for eight hours and then fasting for the remaining sixteen hours.

Some argue that this strategy aids the body's circadian rhythm, or Internal clock, to work more effectively.

Most people can fast at night and for a portion of the day on the 16:8 diet.

Both in the morning and evening, they consume the majority of their calories during the day.

There are no restrictions on the types or quantities of meals consumed throughout the 8-hour interval.

It could be eaten. Because of the simplicity of the strategy, it is relatively easy to implement this adaptability.

How to Go About It

The best way to stay on track with the 16:8 diet is to find a 16-hour fasting window that works for you.

Sleep time is included.

Some doctors advise finishing your meal early in the evening because after that, your metabolism slows down. This is not, however, something that everyone can do.

Some others will be unable to eat until after 7 p.m. or later in the evening. Even then, before going to bed, you should fast for 2–3 hours.

People should eat during one of the eight-hour times listed below:

- Monday through Friday, 9 a.m. to 5 p.m.
- Monday through Friday, 10 a.m. to 6 p.m.
- 12 p.m. to 8 p.m.

During this time, people will eat their meals and snacks whenever they like.

Timeframe. It is critical to eat daily to avoid blood sugar peaks and falls. a voracious appetite experimenting to find out when is the best time to eat and the best time to eat.

For some people, a certain way of living is necessary.

2.20:4

The "One Meal a Day Diet," also known as the "20/4 Diet," is a more extreme version of the "One Meal a Day Diet."

Intermittent fasting is a type of intermittent fasting. The OMAD diet requires people to fast for 23 hours a day.

Allowing them to eat within a one-hour window calorie counting is not part of the OMAD diet.

This diet allows you to eat anything you want, and there are no things that you can't eat. Nutrient-dense diets, are, on the other hand, encouraged for weight loss and overall health.

Many individuals believe that intermittent fasting 20/4 implies restricting one's eating window to just four hours per day. Although this is essentially what a 20-hour fast entails, many people are unaware that Ori Hofmekler, the diet's creator, was a Holocaust survivor.

Mapped out a three-week, three-phase strategy.

According to Ori, this strategy and its phases are critical since they assist you in achieving your goals.

Body to adapt to the Warrior Diet and increase its fat-burning capacity.

The following is the strategy:

Phase One – Week One

The detoxification stage is commonly referred to as this. Ori was involved in this procedure suggests that you:

1. Eat only hard-boiled eggs, yogurt, and healthy grains throughout the 20-hour fast window.

Fruits and vegetables, as well as cottage cheese, are examples of foods that should be consumed.

While you're undereating, consume in small amounts. You are welcome to drink milk.

As for drinks, broth or vegetable juices are acceptable, but only in small quantities. Coffee, tea, and water all of these beverages are enjoyable.

2. The Overeating Window — According to Hofmekler, a salad with oil is the best way to avoid overeating.

During these four hours, you can have a salad with vinegar dressing to break your fast. Following that, you must.

Depending on how much you weigh, you should eat one large meal or a series of smaller ones.

You have a limited amount of time. Beans, whole grains, and other plant-based proteins you may incorporate vegetables into your meals.

Phase Two – Week Two

The "high-fat week" is what it's called. The rules for this phase are as follows:

1. The Undereating Window — During these 20 hours, you can eat the same limited amounts of foods, milk, vegetable juices, and clear broth as you did the first week.

2. The Overeating Window — Unlike the first week, you cannot eat starchy foods, whole grains, or carbohydrates during these four hours. Instead, you'll break your fast with an oil-and-vinegar salad, followed by nuts, cooked veggies, and animal protein for your next meal (or smaller meals).

Phase Three – Week Three

This is known as the "high-carb high-protein cycle" or "concluding fat loss week." This week's nutritional consumption should be as follows:

- 1-2 days high in carbs
- 1-2 days high in protein and low in carbs
- 1-2 days high in carbohydrates
- 1-2 days high in protein and low in carbs
- 1-2 days high in carbohydrates

- 1-2 days high in protein and low in carbs

Days with a lot of carbs

1. Undereating window - Keep eating the same meals as you did the first week.

2. Overeating window — Eat a salad identical to the one you've been eating to break your fast. The next big meal or smaller meals can be made up of some animal protein, some cooked vegetables, and one principal source of carbohydrates: corn, potatoes, rice, barley, whole-wheat pasta, or oats.

Low-Carb – High-Protein Days

1. Consume the same meals and beverages you've been eating and drinking for the past two weeks during the 20-hour underfeeding window.

2. 4-hour Overfeeding Window — Start your day with the same salad, then eat 227 to 454 grams of total animal protein and some no starchy, cooked veggies for the rest of the day.

3. Fruit - While grains and starchy vegetables should be avoided these days, if you're still hungry at the end of the day, consume some fruit.

After the 3-week period has passed, you must start the process all over again.

If you don't like this approach, follow the undereating instructions for the first 20 hours and consume balanced, high-protein meals solely during the 4-hour overfeeding window.

3. 12:12 hours

12:12 is a type of intermittent fasting (IF), a way of eating in which the body burns fat for energy rather than glucose. You are constrained to eating your typical calorie consumption within a 12-hour window and then fasting for the remaining 12 hours, rather than eating whenever you want during the day. This means that if you have dinner at 8 p.m., you won't be ready for breakfast until 8 a.m. the next day. The IF 12:12 is regarded to be the most straightforward.

4. 23:1 (OMAD)

Said, OMAD is the habit of only eating one meal per day. It makes no recommendations as to whether or not you should eat. It only instructs you to eat once. OMAD, equal to a 23:1 easy ratio, is the most extensive form of time-restricted eating (eating in a 1-hour and fasting for 23 hours' window). In its purest form, OMAD does not require calorie restriction or a specific macronutrient structure. Nonetheless, for that meal, it is recommended that you keep to your balanced, low-carb diet.

By combining time-restricted eating and intermittent fasting, OMAD can help regulate diabetes, reduce hyperinsulinemia, and improve metabolic syndrome.

According to clinical practice, expanding the fasting window will exacerbate some metabolic conditions. As a result, OMAD can offer better benefits than shorter fasts when properly practiced.

An example of a week utilizing OMAD is as follows:

- **Monday:** consume 1,800 calories in a 16:8 time-restricted eating pattern by eating two meals.
- **Tuesday:** OMAD (about 1,200 calories) (assuming a daily calorie consumption of 1,800). Aim for a carbohydrate intake of 10 grams, a protein intake of 105 grams, and a fat intake of 104 grams. For some, this amount of information may be overwhelming. If that's the case, try extending your feeding time so you can have a "snack" of nuts and cheese before eating the rest of your meal an hour later.
- **Wednesday:** consume 1,800 calories in two meals following a 16:8 time-restricted eating pattern.
- **Thursday:** as on Tuesday
- **Friday:** 1,800 calories, two meals, and a 16:8 time-restricted diet
- **Saturday:** eat whatever you want (as long as you stay on track with your low-carb diet!)
- **Sunday:** identical to Tuesday

5. 5:2

The 5:2 diet gets its name because it regularly eats five days a week and severely reduces food consumption on the other two.

Although the name "fasting" is a little misleading, the 5:2 diet is a popular kind of intermittent fasting.

Unlike a truly fast, which involves going without meals for a set amount of time, the 5:2 diet aims to keep calorie intake on fasting days to 25% of total daily intake on non-fasting days.

An individual who regularly consumes 2,000 calories per day will consume 500 calories on fasting days.

It is necessary to provide the body with the calories and nutrients it needed to thrive, and fasting days do not have to be consecutive.

Fasting days are generally alternated, such as Mondays and Thursdays or Wednesdays and Saturdays.

Part of the diet's allure is its versatility. Instead of strictly restricting a person's food intake, the 5:2 diet emphasizes strict nutritional management on just two days of the week. Certain people will feel more at ease with their food due to this, and they will not feel deprived all of the time.

On the five regular days of the 5:2 diet, however, a nutritious diet should be followed.

It's possible that bingeing on processed or sugary meals for five days and then taking a break won't be as successful as sticking to a clean eating regimen during the week.

The 5:2 diet has many advantages, including weight loss and a reduced risk of type 2 diabetes.

Include foods in your diet.

- fiber and vegetables
- a source of protein
- berries that are dark in color

Foods to stay away from

- processed foods, which are often refined and heavy in calories.
- saturated fats, such as those found in animal fats, cooking oils, and cheese.
- refined carbohydrate foods like pasta, bread, and white rice

6. Fasting on alternate days

Intermittent fasting can take several forms, including alternate-day fasting.

You can fast any day you like on this diet, but you can eat whatever you want on non-fasting days.

The most popular variation of this diet is "modified" fasting, which permits you to eat.

On fasting days, roughly 500 calories are consumed.

Fasting on alternate days can help you lose weight while also increasing your risk of heart disease.

Type 2 diabetes and kidney failure are two conditions that can lead to death.

For novices, here's a step-by-step introduction to alternate-day fasting.

ADF's potential advantages by the end of the research period, the ADF had earned some advantages, including which have been related to a longer life span

- Body weight and belly fat have both decreased.
- Ketone levels have risen.
- A biological marker's levels have dropped.
- Cholesterol levels are lower.

What is the mechanism behind it?

On fasting days, you can drink as many calorie-free beverages as you want. Here are several examples:

Here are several examples:

- the element of water
- a cup of tea

- coffee that is not sweetened

You must ingest approximately 500 calories each day, or 20–25 percent of your total daily calories.

If you're utilizing a modified ADF approach, you'll require more energy on fasting days.

Dr. Krista Varady, who has conducted the majority of the ADF research, has named the most.

The "Every Other Day Diet" is a popular variation of this diet.

Whether the fasting-day calories are consumed around lunch or supper, or in little amounts throughout the day, the benefits of eating meals during the day on wellbeing and weight loss appear to be the same.

For some people, alternate-day fasting is easier to maintain than other types of fasting of different diets commitment to alternate-day fasting (in which calorie consumption is restricted on alternate days), on the other hand, on fasting days, limited to 25% of calorie requirements) was not preferred to daily calorie restriction during a year.

Most diets now incorporate an updated version of 500 calories on fasting days.

Fasting on alternate days is an experiment. This is anticipated to be far more long-term.

It is less successful than total fasts on fasting days, but it is still effective.

7. Longer fasts

A 48-hour fast is the most common length of time for protracted fasting.

In principle, a 48-hour fast is simple: you give yourself a two-day vacation from eating.

On the first day, one popular strategy is to avoid eating after dinner.

On the third day, you can resume eating.

Zero-calorie beverages such as black coffee, water, and tea should also be consumed contrary to popular perception, during the fasting period drink plenty of water to avoid dehydration, which is one of the most dangerous side effects.

during extended fasting periods following that, it's critical to reintroduce meals gradually. As a result, the overstimulated stomach, which can lead to nausea, bloating, and other unpleasant symptoms as well as diarrhea your first meal should be a light snack, such as a handful or two of almonds.

The famine A light meal should be served one or two hours later.

You can eat regularly on non-fasting days, as long as you don't overeat in calorie-dense meals it's more common to do a 48-hour fast once or twice a month rather than every day.

Most fasting methods call for fasting once or twice a week. It's not impossible.

Further health benefits can be obtained by properly spacing out the 48-hour fasts.

Fasting for 48 hours is not recommended for everyone, so try shorter fasts first.

Before committing to a two-day session, as the 16:8 or alternate-day approaches.

This will help you understand how the body reacts to a nutritional change.

1.5 Tips and Tricks to Make the Most Out of Intermittent Fasting.

If you decide to utilize IF, it has a lot of best for dieting, especially if you're attempting to lose weight because that's when I find IF most effective.

When done correctly, it can assist you;

Allowing yourself to eat larger meals once you do eat can help you manage hunger.

Allowing you more nutritional flexibility can help you stick to your diet.

When it comes to overall success and capacity to attain your goals, managing hunger & sticking to the diet is critical. Intermittent fasting may help you achieve this, but while some people may fast for lengthy periods with minimal difficulty, others, especially when first starting out, may find it more challenging.

Here are some suggestions to help you get the most from your time & make the journey a little simpler.

1: Begin your fast right after dinner.

One of the finest ideas I can give you will be to start your fasting after dinner if you're undertaking daily or weekly fasts. This implies you'll sleep for the majority of your fasting period. Especially if you use a daily fasting schedule like 16:8 and begin fasting after dinner.

Spend 1–3 hours watching television or engaging in other evening activities.

Sleep for 6 to 9 hours.

You've previously fasted for 7–12 hours, which makes a 16-hour fast much more bearable. That is to say; increased commitment to a healthy diet a more relaxed way of living hunger is easier to control is Skipping Breakfast Dangerous for Your Health?

2: Consume More Satisfying Foods

Every food you eat has an impact on your ability to stick to the diet and fast, & this is where IF may assist you out. Consider your typical fat-loss diet:

In the morning, have eggs or porridge.

A tasteless lunch of unrefined chicken breast, sweet potato, and vegetables followed.

After your workout, eat some protein and drink some water or a milkshake.

Then you end the day with a similarly uninspired evening meal.

If you're lucky, you'll be able to scrounge up enough calories to eat a handful of nuts a few times a day. You're dissatisfied and dissatisfied with the prospect of having to start all over again, & again, and again, until you reach your goal weight...if you don't stop first.

Not to add the hunger and desires that come with a diet like this. Consider your fat-loss diet when you're fasting intermittently.

You forego breakfast in favor of water & coffee (and any other calorie-free beverage – see #4).

Lunchtime arrives, and you're still eating chicken breast, but this time it's seasoned with a fantastic BBQ sauce and served with creamy potatoes & a side of vegetables with dressing.

After your workout, eat some protein and drink some water or a milkshake.

It's dinnertime, and you're out celebrating a friend's birthday with pizza.

This would have made you panic out or, worse, not show up since you didn't would like to mess up your metabolism; however, with the calorie saved by skipping breakfast, you take your part and know you're still inside your daily calorie allowance.

You have more than enough calories that included 1–2 little snacks on days when you aren't out in the evening omelet.

This sets IF apart from other dietary protocols: the ability to eat whatever foods you choose and consume a more gratifying and so satiating diet. Foods that are satiating include:

- Potatoes
- Yogurt
- Eggs
- Bananas
- Oatmeal
- Soups

Or items that you can consume in large quantities without eating a large number of calories;

- Fruits
- Vegetables
- Legumes

This isn't an excuse to binge (see point #2), but it is an opportunity to design a fat-loss diet that you will love and stick to in the long run.

3: Maintain a busy schedule

Boredom is your adversary. It's the silent murderer that quietly eats away at your progress, gradually wearing you down to pull you backward. Consider this for a moment...

How often has boredom caused you to eat more than you should want or even know you are doing?

You're at work doing something monotonous, and the snacks that have been allowed into the kitchen call to you.

You're at the house watching Netflix, which is fine but not very engaging, and you catch yourself reaching for the munchies mindlessly.

You're in the airport, waiting for your flight, and you're exploring the shops or sitting in restaurants...eating.

But what exactly makes you eat when you're bored?

This is due to dopamine, a neurotransmitter found in the brain. Dopamine is important for reward-motivated behavior and makes you feel good when you achieve a goal.

Eating has been shown to boost glucose levels and, as a result, the positive feelings it produces. More than that, it's 'junk food that makes you feel terrific, especially foods heavy in sugar, fat, & sodium.

Existing research (1) demonstrates that individuals who were boring ate more calories than those that are not bored, and a new study (2, 3) reveals that "boredom markedly increases food intake [in] either obese and normal [subjects]."

It's hardly strange that you eat more than when you're bored; your brain is almost programmed to seek out that dopamine is high.

How and when to Stick to A Diet Without Going Off the Rails

4: Suppress Your Appetite

When fasting, hunger sensations may undoubtedly strike from time to time. When this occurs, the key is to suppress your appetite, and the correct method to do it is with zero-calorie liquids that assist produce fullness and hold cravings at bay until your fast is broken.

You're good to go as long because as a drink has no calories; examples include:

- Water
- Water that sparkles
- A cup of black coffee
- A cup of black tea
- Green tea is a type of tea that is used.
- Diet beverages

5: Eat A Regular-Sized Meal to Break Your Fast

When we discussed how IF isn't an excuse to consume everything you want, we mentioned this. Provided, like any other diet, only effective for fat reduction or muscle gain if you maintain sufficient calorie deficits. This implies when it is an opportunity to remove your fast, you don't want to take any chances, especially if your goal is to lose weight.

Yes, skipping breakfast saves calories and allows you to eat more at other times, but if you go too far, you'll destroy the calorie deficit that you worked so hard to achieve. Now, the amount of your meal upon breaking the fast will be determined by whether you just finished working out or will be working out later throughout the day.

With that in mind, here are a few pointers to help you stay on track:

1 – I've Only Just Worked Out

In this situation, this meal should account for 50–60% of your total calories and comprise various macronutrients.

2 – Exercising Later

In this case, you would like this meal to account for 30–50% of your total calories, and it should contain a variety of macronutrients.

These tips will assist you in breaking your fast sans going overboard by providing an estimate about how much to consume based upon your circumstances.

You'll get the most out of your fast if you get this phase right, as you'll be able to maintain the proper calorie intake while still having enough calories to enjoy satisfying meals late in the day.

6: Sticking to a Schedule

The Cambridge Dictionary defines routine as "a normal or fixed way of doing business," and when it comes to HOW this may be accomplished, it may be done through;

Every day, start and end your fast at the same time.

Following a weekly diet that consists of the same (or comparable) foods each day preparing food ahead of time it's easier to stay to your IF plan if you have a routine. When you figure out what works for both of you and adhere to it every day, you eliminate hesitation and third. All you can do now is carry it out.

Not to mention that sticking to a regimen reduces decision fatigue. Which is the phrase for when your capacity to make decisions deteriorates after a long period of making them. This indicates that if you're constantly faced with decisions such as;

What you're going to eat?

When are you going to eat it?

When you have the opportunity to prepare it?

If the calories and macros are right for you, go for it.

You'll ultimately reach a point where your "decision-making muscle" is worn down, and you'll make the erroneous or easy decision. By lowering the number, the decisions, you have to make each day, you're effectively removing potential roadblocks to your success.

If you're having trouble making the results you desire and frequently find yourself deviating from your diet & fasting hours, setting up a schedule will help.

7: Allow time for self-adjustment

It's only natural to want immediate results...

To skip the uncomfortable novice stage and get right to a seasoned expert or at the very least the "I kind of know what I'm doing" stage. On the other hand, bypassing this initial learning step is to set oneself up for failure. Fasting requires time for your body to acclimatize, especially if it is your first day.

It's very normal to experience hunger pangs before you even begin, and it's also very reasonable to make a few mistakes. This does not imply that you should give up nor that it will not work for you. Instead, it's a chance to learn, to ponder why or how you made a mistake, and to take action to prevent it from happening again.

You will be aware of future issues as a result of going through this process.

Trust this process and stick with it even when things become tough; remember that no one is great the first time, the tenth time, or even the hundredth time; persist with it, and you'll not only adjust, but you'll also be taking the very first step toward developing the attitude you have to succeed.

8: Have the Right Attitude

I know I sound dumb, but the most crucial ideas frequently need to be read several times before they truly sink in. It's one of those instances... If nothing is working for you, skipping breakfast is not a quick fix or a shortcut to your goals.

It's just another nutritional option that can be quite beneficial to some people when taken correctly and under one's lifestyle. It's vital to remember this when using IF and understand that these results are entirely dependent on you though it can provide amazing outcomes.

Keeping track of your calorie & macronutrient intake

Consistent training

Overloading the system gradually.

This is true for all diets, so whether you're doing intermittent fasting or something else, bear that in mind. Here are three strategies to help you develop this mindset:

Set goals based on what's truly achievable, not really what you wished was achievable.

Be laser-focused in your efforts & understand that the best path to success is to put in persistent work toward a single goal.

Be patient and understand that as you didn't lose your dream physique in a day, week, or month, you won't be able to reclaim it in the same time frame.

9: Consume BCAAs

When training while fasting, you should ingest 10 grams of BCAAs (branched-chain amino acids) when you begin.

If you're not going to break your fast after your workout, it's a good idea to take extra 10 grams. However, if you time your first meal after your workout, you won't need to worry about the next dosage.

10: Have a good time

Intermittent fasting, when done correctly, can afford significant nutritional freedom and thus happiness. This is because, depending about what you regularly eat, skipping breakfast can save you anywhere from 300 to 1,000 calories.

To make your diet more enjoyable, you can move these calories to your lunch, supper, or 1–2 snacks. As an example;

Dinner for a friend's birthday in the evening? It's no problem! Skip breakfast in favor of a protein-rich lunch, and you'll have enough calories you enjoy in the evening without exceeding your daily calorie limit.

Are you planning a vacation or a trip? Great! Skip breakfast, get plenty of exercises, and eat two large meals each afternoon and evening.

Do you have a calorie deficit? Sure! Stop eating breakfast to save calories that could be utilized to eat more filling meals late in the day avoid constantly feeling hungry while attempting to lose weight.

Is there any other form of social gathering? Have fun with it! You may always conserve calories by fasting for any occasion where you expect to eat much more usual.

Of course, you should still follow the 70/30 guideline (also known as the 60/40 / 80/20 rule), which states that the bulk of your diet should consist of nutritious foods containing a diverse mix of minerals and vitamins, as well as a variety of macronutrients. The remaining 30% can be made up of foods you enjoy, even whether they lack minerals and vitamins. As a result of this, you will be able to:

Maintain your sanity.

Attempt to avoid urges.

Maintain your diet.

Point of Sale

IF is a fantastic dietary strategy for reducing weight, and while some people seem to fly through their fast even without thinking about eating, others find it more difficult.

A little assistance might go a way away in assisting these individuals in getting the most of quickly. If you follow the guidelines outlined in this section, you would be able to do just that;

- Defend yourself against hunger
- When you're hungry, don't eat blindly.
- Keep your eating habits in check.
- Maintain your diet.

1.6 Common mistakes people do when approaching intermittent fasting.

1. Getting started quickly with intermittent fasting

One of the biggest blunders you can make is to start too quickly. You can set oneself up for failure if you plunge into IF without first easing into it. It can be not easy to transition from eating three large meals or six little meals a day to eating inside a four-hour timeframe, for example.

Instead, gradually introduce fasting. If you want to use the 16/8 approach, gradually increase the duration between meals till you can work comfortably in 12 hours. Then, to get the window down to 8 hours, subtract a few minutes a day when you're there.

2. Choosing the wrong intermittent fasting plan

You've bought entire foods like fish & chicken, fruits and vegetables, and nutritious sides like quinoa & lentils, and you're ready to attempt Intermittent Fasting in weight loss. The issue is that you haven't chosen the IF strategy that will ensure your success. For example, if you go to the gym six days a week, fully fasting over two of those days might not be the best approach for you.

Rather than jumping into a program without thinking about it, examine your lifestyle and choose the plan that best suits your schedule and habits.

3. Excessive eating in the fasting window

The shorter time left to eat means ingesting fewer calories, which is one reason many choose to attempt Intermittent Fasting. On the other hand, some folks will eat their typical number of calories during the fasting window. Therefore, it's possible that you won't lose weight as a result of this.

Don't eat your daily calorie intake of 2000 calories within a window. Instead, aim for a caloric intake of 1200 - 1500 calories at the time you're breaking the fast. Whether you fast for 4, 6, and 8 hours, the number of meals that you eat will also be determined by the length of a fasting window. If you find yourself in a state of poverty and need to eat, reassess the plan you selected to follow, or take a day off the IF to focus and then go back on track.

4. In your fasting window, eating the wrong food items

Overeating coincides with the Interval Training mistake from eating the incorrect things. You will not feel well if you have a fasting period of 6 hours and fill this with processed, fatty, or sugary foods.

As I mentioned in my piece, Eating Clean for Beginners, eat healthy whole foods. The mainstay of your diet becomes lean proteins, good fats, nuts, legumes, unprocessed grains, and healthful vegetables and fruits. In addition, when you're not fasting, keep these healthy dietary suggestions in mind:

Rather than eating at a restaurant, cook & eat at home.

Read nutrition labels to learn about additives like corn syrup & modified palm oil that aren't allowed.

Keep an eye out for hidden sweeteners and limit your sodium intake.

Instead of manufactured foods, cook whole foods.

Fiber, nutritious carbs and fats, & lean proteins should all be present in your meal.

5. Calorie restriction in the fasting window

Yes, there is such thing as calorie restriction that is excessive. It's not healthy to eat or less than 1200 calories during your fasting window. Not just that, but it has the potential to slow down your metabolic rate. If you reduce your metabolism too much, you'll start losing muscle mass instead of gaining it.

To avoid making this error, plan your meals for the week forward on the weekend. You'll have balanced, healthful meals at your fingertips in no time. Then, when it's time to eat, one can choose from various healthful, nutritional, and calorie-balanced options.

6. Breaking an intermittent fast without realizing it

It's important to be mindful of hidden quick breakers. For example, did you guys know that the taste of sugar makes your brain release insulin? This triggers the release of insulin, thereby breaking the fast. Here is some unexpected food, supplements, & products that can stop a fast and trigger an insulin response:

Supplements containing malt dextrin and pectin, as well as other ingredients

Sugar and fat are found in vitamins like gummy bear vitamins.

Using toothpaste & mouthwash with xylitol as a sweetener

Sugar can be found in the coating of pain medicines like Advil.

Breaking your fast is a common Intermittent Fasting blunder. When you're not eating, clean your teeth with a baking soda & water paste, read the instructions carefully and take vitamins & supplements.

7. Drinking insufficiently during intermittent fasting

IF necessitates that you stay hydrated. Keep in mind that your body isn't absorbing the fluids that would normally be eaten with the meal. As a result, if you're not careful, adverse effects can throw you off. For example, if you allow yourself to become dehydrated, you may have headaches, muscle cramps, & severe hunger.

Also include following in your day to avoid this mistake & avoid unpleasant symptoms like cramping & headaches:

Water

2 tbsp. apple cider vinegar and water

a cup of black coffee

Green tea, black tea, herbal tea, oolong tea, or oolong tea

8. When intermittently fasting, do not exercise

Some people believe they can't exercise during an IF period when in reality, it's the ideal situation. Exercising helps you burn fat that has been stored in your body. Additionally, while you exercise, your Human Growth Hormone levels rise, assisting in muscular growth. There are, however, some guidelines to follow to get the most out of your workouts.

Keep the following factors in mind to receive the best outcomes from your efforts:

Time your workouts to coincide with meal times, and then consume nutritious carbs & proteins in 30 minutes after finishing your workout.

If the workout is strenuous, make sure that you eat beforehand to replenish your glycogen stores.

Base your workout on your fasting approach; if you're fasting for 24 hours, don't do anything strenuous that day.

During the fast, and particularly during the workout, stay hydrated.

Pay attention to your body's signals; if you start to feel faint or light-headed, relax or stop working out.

9. Being too strict on yourself when intermittently fasting if you slip

One blunder does not equal defeat! You'll have days whenever an IF diet is especially difficult, and you don't believe you'll be able to keep up. It's quite ok to take breaks if necessary. Set aside a day to focus. Stick to your healthy eating plan, but indulge in delights like an excellent protein shake or a portion of nutritious beef and broccoli the next day.

Don't fall into the trap of letting Intermittent Fasting take over your entire life. Instead, consider it a part of a healthy lifestyle, and don't forget to take care of yourself in other ways. Enjoy a good book, get some exercise, spend quality time with your family, & eat as healthy as possible. It's all part of the process of becoming the best version of yourself.

Chapter 2: How to Begin with Intermittent Fasting

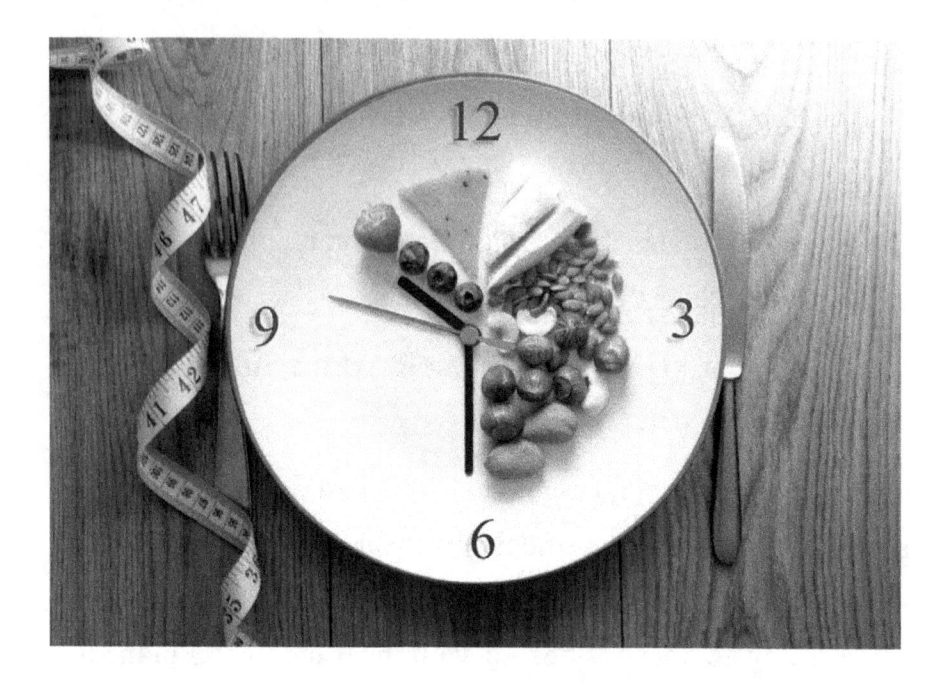

It's important to note that intermittent fasting is not really a diet. It is a method of eating that is timed. Unlike a dietary plan that limits where calories originate from, intermittent fasting does not define which items a person should consume or avoid. Although intermittent fasting has various health benefits, notably weight loss, it is not for everyone.

Intermittent fasting entails alternating between eating and fasting times. Women may find it challenging at first to eat only for a short period of time each day or to alternate between eating & not eating days. In this chapter, you will get advice on getting started fasting, such as setting personal goals, preparing meals, and determining caloric requirements.

Intermittent fasting is a famous approach for achieving the following goals:

- make their lives simplify
- weight loss
- minimize the consequences of aging, and increase their general health and well-being

Fasting is generally safe for the healthiest, well-nourished women. However, it may not be acceptable for those with medical issues. The following guidelines are intended to assist individuals who are ready to begin fasting in making it as simple & successful as possible.

2.1 Determine your Personal objectives.

A person who begins intermittent fasting usually has a specific purpose in mind. It could be for weight loss, better general health, or better metabolic health. A person's ultimate aim will aid them in determining the best fasting strategy and calculating how many calories & nutrients they require.

2.2 Select a method.

Before attempting another fasting strategy, a person should usually stick with one for at least a month.

When it comes to fasting for health reasons, there are four options to consider. First, a person should choose the strategy that best meets their needs and believe they will keep to.

These are some of them:

- Eat stop & eat
- Diet of the Warrior &
- Leangains
- Fasting on alternate days

Before adopting a different fasting strategy, a person should usually continue with one for a full month to discover if it works for them. In addition, before commencing any fasting program, anyone with a medical issue should consult their doctor.

When choosing a strategy, keep in mind that you don't have to eat a certain quantity or type of food or avoid some meals entirely. A person is free to consume whatever they desire. However, it is good to consume a healthy, high-fiber, vegetable-rich diet to achieve health and weight loss goals during the eating periods.

On eating days, bingeing on unhealthy meals might sabotage your health. During the fast days, it's also critical to drink enough water or other low-calorie liquids.

2.2.1 Eat Stop & Eat

Eat Brad Pilon created stop Eat, and it is a fasting approach that entails not eating for 24 hours twice a week. It makes no difference how many days a woman fasts or when they begin. The only stipulation is that fasting must be done for at least 24 hours & on separate days.

Women who go without eating for more than 24 hours are prone to get really hungry. Eat Stop Eat might not be the best technique for folks who are new to fasting.

2.2.2 Diet of the Warrior

The Warrior Diet, created by Ori Hofmekler, comprises eating little to nothing for 20 hours each day. In the remaining four hours, individuals fasting in this manner consumes all of their usual food consumption.

Eating a whole day's worth of meals can upset a person's stomach in such a short period of time. That's the most intense fasting strategy, and like Eat Stop Eat, it is not recommended for someone who is new to fasting.

2.2.3 Leangains

Martin Berkhan designed Leangains for weightlifters, but it has since gained appeal among other people interested in fasting. Fasting for Leangains is substantially shorter than it is for Eat Stop Eat & the Warrior Diet.

Females over 50 who pick the Leangains approach, for example, will fast for around 14 hours and afterward eat whatever they need for the next 10 hours.

During the fast, one must refrain from eating any food but may consume as many non-calorie beverages as desired

2.2.4 5:2 method of alternate-day fasting

To enhance blood sugar, cholesterol, & weight loss, some individuals fast on alternate days. For example, on the 5:2 diet, a person consumes 500 to 600 calories on two non-consecutive days per week.

Some alternate-day fasting plans include a third fasting day each week. A person eats only the amount of calories they expend during the day for the remainder of the week. This results in a calorie deficit over time, allowing the person to lose weight.

Online resources are accessible for the Warrior, Eat Stop Eat, & Leangains fasting methods.

2.3 Determine your calorie requirements

When fasting, there are no food limitations, but calories must still be counted.

People who want to lose weight must develop a calorie deficit, which means they must consume fewer calories than they expend. Conversely, those who want to acquire weight must take in more calories than they expend.

Numerous tools are available to assist a person in calculating their caloric requirements and determining how several calories they must take each day to lose or gain weight. A person could also seek advice from a healthcare physician or a dietitian about the number of calories they require.

2.4 Create a meal plan.

A person who is trying to lose or gain weight may find that planning their meals for the day or week is beneficial.

Meal preparation does not have to be limiting. Instead, it considers calorie intake and ensures that the right nutrients are included in the diet.

Meal planning has several advantages, including assisting with calorie counting and ensuring that a person has the appropriate supplies on hand for cooking dishes, quick meals, & snacks.

2.5 Keep track of your calories.

Calories aren't all created equal. Although these fasting methods do not specify the number of calories a person should take when fasting, the meal's nutritional value must be considered.

In general, nutrient-dense food, or the food with both a high amount of nutrients per calorie, should be consumed. However, even if a person does not have to avoid junk food completely, they should still eat it in moderation & focus on healthier alternatives to reap the greatest benefits.

2.6 Exercise-related effects

Intermittent fasting must not influence the capacity to exercise in women over 50, save during the time when the body adjusts to the new eating pattern. A person should not experience any negative impacts from fasting on their workout habit after the adjustment period.

Those concerned about muscle loss during fasting should ingest enough protein during feeding periods and engage in regular resistance training. Fasting is less likely to cause muscle loss if protein consumption is maintained.

Chapter 3: Intermittent Fasting Health Benefits for Women Over 50

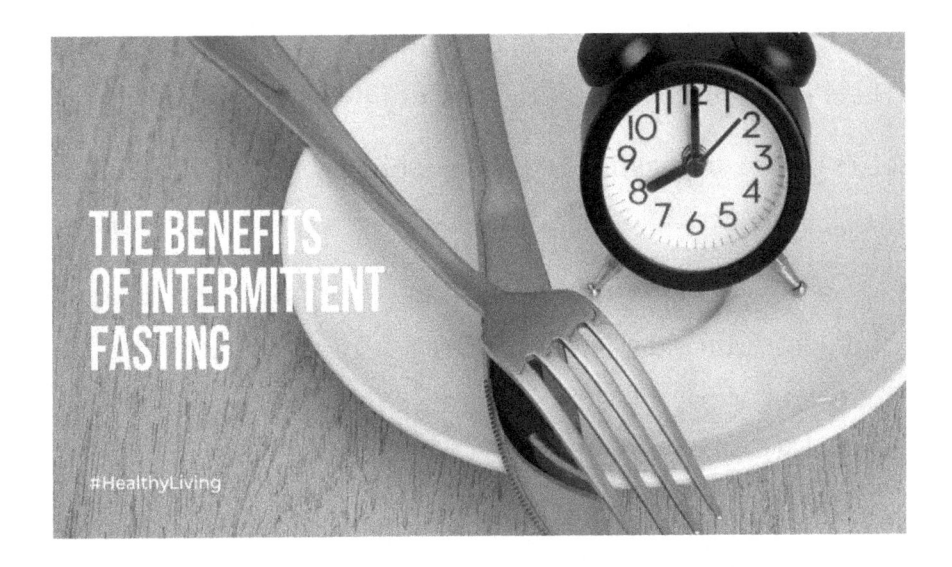

(IF) can help you lose weight while also lowering your risk of acquiring various chronic conditions.

3.1 Cardiovascular Health

The main death cause in the world is heart disease.

High blood pressure, higher LDL cholesterol, and high triglyceride levels are three of the most common factors for heart disease.

Intermittent fasting for women over 50 reduced blood pressure by 6% in about eight weeks in a study of 16 obese men and women.

According to the same study, intermittent fasting also reduced LDL cholesterol by 25% & triglycerides by 32%.

So, evidence suggesting a relationship between intermittent fasting and lower LDL cholesterol & triglyceride levels is mixed.

4 weeks of the intermittent fasting, as during the Islamic holiday of Ramadan, showed no result in a reduction in LDL cholesterol or triglycerides, according to a study of 40 normal-weight per.

Before researchers can fully comprehend the impact of intermittent fasting on heart health, higher-quality studies with much more robust techniques are required.

3.2 Diabetes

Intermittent fasting can also help you control your diabetes and lower your chance of developing it.

Intermittent fasting, like continuous calorie restriction, appears to lower several diabetes risks factors.

It primarily accomplishes this by reducing insulin levels and decreasing insulin resistance.

Six months of intermittent fasting lowered insulin levels by 29% & insulin resistance by 19% in a randomized control study of more than around 100 overweight or obese women. The blood lactate levels were unchanged.

Furthermore, (IF) for 8–12 weeks has been proven to lower glucose levels by 20–31% & blood lactate levels by 3–6% in people with anti-diabetes, a situation in which blood lactate levels are high but not strong enough to diagnose diabetes.

In terms of blood sugar, though, (IF) may not be quite as good for women as it is for men.

A tiny study indicated that women's blood sugar management deteriorated after 22 days of the alternate-day fasting, whereas men's blood sugar levels were unaffected.

Given this side effect, the decrease in insulin & insulin resistance would certainly minimize the risk of diabetes, especially in anti-diabetic persons.

3.3 Loss of weight

When done correctly, intermittent fasting could be a simple and successful strategy to reduce weight, as short-term fasts can assist you to consume fewer calories and lose weight.

Several studies have found that intermittent fasting is just as successful as typical calorie-restricted diets for weight loss in the short term.

Intermittent fasting resulted in average losing weight of 15 lbs. (6.8 kg) over 3–12 months, according to a 2018 review of trials in overweight persons.

According to another study for 3–24 weeks, intermittent fasting lowered body weight by 3–8% in overweight or obese people. According to the study, participants lowered their waist size by 3–7% during the same period.

It's worth noting that the long-term consequences of intermittent fasting on female weight loss are still unknown.

Intermittent fasting appears to help with weight loss in the short term. However, the quantity you lose will most likely be determined by how many calories you take during non-fasting periods & also how long you stick to the diet.

3.4 It Might Assist You in Eating Less

Turning to intermittent fasting can help you eat less naturally.

According to one study, when young men's food consumption was confined to a four-hour timeframe, they ate 650 fewer calories each day.

Another study looked at the impact of a long, 36-hour fast on dietary behaviors in 24 healthy men & women. Despite eating more calories on the post-fast day, individuals' total calorie balance reduced by 1,900 calories, a considerable decrease.

3.5 Fat-burning and Noradrenaline

Fasting causes your nervous system to send out neurotransmitter messages (noradrenaline) that cause your body to burn fat for energy. As a result, the procedure leads to a long-term weight decrease without sacrificing muscular mass.

3.6 Defend Against Oxidative Stress

Multiple age-related illnesses are exacerbated by oxidative stress (unstable chemicals that destroy cells). According to research, IF can help you boost your biological defenses against free radicals.

3.7 Increases Life Expectancy

As per Harvard study, IF can change the function of mitochondria (energy-producing organelles in cells) and perhaps lengthen life spans. Fasting has been shown to flip mitochondrial networks, keeping them young and promoting fat metabolism.

3.8 Other Health Advantages

Intermittent fasting may potentially have various health benefits, according to several animal and human research.

- Intermittent fasting has been shown in several studies to lower major markers of inflammation. Chronic inflammation can cause weight gain and a slew of other health issues.

- Improved psychological well-being: According to one study, 8 weeks of intermittent fasting reduced depression & binge eating behaviors in obese people while enhancing body image.

- Maintain muscle mass: Compared to constant calorie restriction, intermittent fasting appears to be much more successful at retaining muscle mass. Even while you're at rest, having more muscle mass assists, you burn more calories.

Before any judgments can be formed about the benefits of intermittent fasting for women, additional research needs to be done in well-designed human studies.

Chapter 4: How Intermittent Fasting Works for Women Over 50

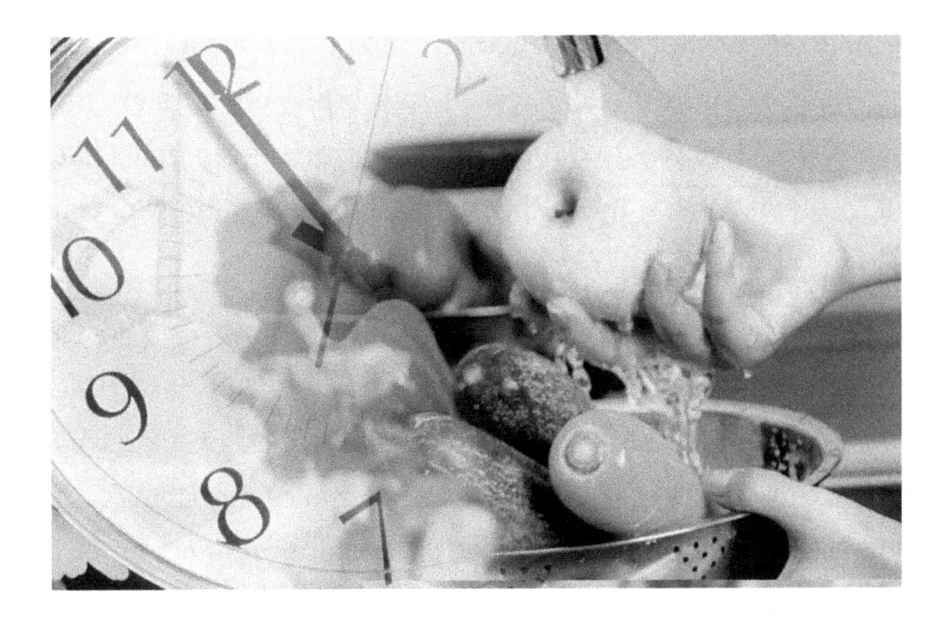

The basic goal of intermittent fasting is to redirect the body's attention away from food digestion and toward things like recuperation and maintenance. During the fasting phase, your body effectively enters into starvation mode & through a number of metabolic changes. Because there is no food in the stomach to digest, the body concentrates on recuperation and maintenance. Second, when carbs are unavailable, the body enters ketosis, a state during which stored fat in the body is consumed for energy. This procedure aids in weight loss.

Intermittent fasting means simply going without food for a period of time, usually between 12 and 48 hours. Your fasting window is the period of time during which you only ingest liquids such as herbal tea, water or broth.

To help maintain vitamin and mineral intake regular when fasting, some experts suggest drinking low-calorie green vegetable juices & taking supplements, while others feel only water should be ingested. Intermittent fasting regulations, like many other aspects of health, are debatable based on who you ask.

You will have an eating window if you fast for fewer than 24 hours. This is the amount of time you have to eat before starting your fast. The eating window for most women over 50 who practice intermittent fasting is between six and twelve hours. 12 hours, 14 hours, 16 hours, and 18 hours are the most typical fasting times.

If you fasted for 12 hours, for example, you're eating window would indeed be 12 hours. You might begin eating at 7 a.m. and conclude at 7 p.m. The next day, at 7 a.m., you should break the fast.

While some of the intermittent fasting methods available online appear to be more intensive than others (some can go up to 48 hours), the overall beauty of intermittent fasting is that you can choose and experiment with the length of your fast. This allows you to not only figure out how intermittent fasting fits into your lifestyle but also to find the happy fasting medium that makes you feel the best physically.

4.1 Pros and Cons of Intermittent Fasting for Women Over 50 (And Why It Can Get Tricky)

Intermittent fasting may provide the following advantages:

- Weight loss that lasts
- A gain in lean muscle mass
- More vitality
- An increase in the stress response of cells
- Inflammation and oxidative stress are reduced.
- Insulin resistance in overweight women is improved.
- Increased neurotrophic growth factor production (which might boost cognitive function)

Here's when it gets tricky. Although intermittent fasting has some advantages, women are more sensitive to signals of famine than men; therefore, intermittent fasting for women over 50 is a different beast altogether.

When the female body feels that famine is approaching, it increases the production of the appetite hormones ghrelin & leptin, which tell the body that it's time to eat. Furthermore, if you don't have enough nourishment to thrive, your body will shut down the whole system that allows you to generate another human. Even if you're not pregnant or attempting to conceive, this is the body's natural way of protecting a prospective pregnancy.

It's not that you're deliberately starving yourself, but your body isn't aware of this. Because it can't tell the difference between actual starving and intermittent fasting, it falls back on this defensive strategy.

As a result, some of the disadvantages linked with hormonal imbalances caused by intermittent fasting may include:

- Periods that are irregular (or entire loss of period)
- Stress on the metabolism
- The ovaries are shrinking.
- Anxiety
- Sleeping problems

Because all of the hormones are so closely linked, when one is disrupted, the others suffer as well. It's like a chain reaction. You don't want to mess with the "messengers" that control practically every function in your body, from energy production to digestion, metabolism, & blood pressure.

With all of these disadvantages, you might be wondering if you could (or would) practice intermittent fasting as a woman who is over 50. The answer to that is yes if you adopt a more casual approach. Intermittent fasting, when done for a shorter period of time, can still help you lose weight and deliver the other benefits described above without ruining your hormones.

4.2 The Best Intermittent Fasting Techniques for Women Over 50

So, what does it mean to have a laid-back attitude to intermittent fasting? We're dealing with a bit of a murky area here because there hasn't been much significant research on intermittent fasting. The views differ depending on whatever website you visit or which health professional you consult. According to what we've discovered, the general guidelines for women when it comes to brief intermittent fasting are as follows:

- Do not go without food for more than 24 hours at a time.
- Fast for 12 to 16 hours if possible.
- During the first two to three weeks of fasting, avoid fasting on consecutive days (Suppose, if you are doing a 16-hour fast, do it 3 days a week instead of 7)
- During your fast, drink plenty of fluids (like bone broth, herbal tea, or water).
- On fasting days, only conduct light activities such as yoga, jogging, walking, & easy stretching.

Intermittent fasting allows you to eat anything you want. However, this does not grant you the right to have anything you want. You must eat things that are both healthful and nourishing. Even during the fasting window, you must avoid breaking your fast by consuming anything containing calories.

Drinks high in carbohydrates or sugar can cause your body to secrete insulin, preventing you from realizing the rewards of intermittent fasting. What you can eat and drink when fasting:

- Water is a calorie-free beverage that will keeps you hydrated.
- Coffee or tea with barely a teaspoon of milk- Only drink unsweetened tea or coffee.
- Apple Cider Vinegar—Diluted apple cider vinegar might help you stay hydrated and avoid cravings when fasting.

4.3 When Should Intermittent Fasting Be Avoided?

Not everyone is a good fit for intermittent fasting. If you're one of the following women, intermittent fasting isn't a good idea:

- When you're under a lot of pressure,
- History of eating disorders
- Have trouble sleeping

Furthermore, intermittent fasting is supposed to supplement a good diet and lifestyle, not to compensate for five days of eating nutritionally deficient items like processed foods, refined sugar, and fast food.

4.4 Side Effects and Safety

Most women over 50 appear to be safe when using modified variants of intermittent fasting.

On the other hand, a number of studies have found that fasting days might cause hunger, mood changes, lack of concentration, decreased energy, headaches, and foul breath.

Women's menstrual cycles have also been reported to have ceased while on an intermittent fasting diet, according to some reports on the internet.

Before attempting intermittent fasting, ask your doctor if you have a medical issue.

- Medical advice is especially necessary for women who:
- Have an eating disorder history.
- Have diabetes or encounter low blood sugar on a frequent basis.
- Are underweight, malnourished, or deficient in nutrients.
- Have fertility issues or a history of amenorrhea? (missed periods).

Finally, intermittent fasting seems to have a favorable safety profile. However, if you have any issues, such as an absence of your menstrual period, you should stop immediately.

4.5 Tips on Getting Started

It's not easy to adjust to intermittent fasting, especially if you're doing it all at once. One thing we must surely avoid throughout our eating periods is bingeing on big amounts of processed foods. We might not notice any outcomes if we try this! First and foremost, I urge that you change your dietary habits. Before attempting intermittent fasting, getting into a routine of eating as healthily as possible would be quite beneficial. Start doing this two week before you actually plan to start your intermittent fasting regimen, and it will make the adjustment much smoother.

It's challenging to stay on track, but here's what you should do to stay on track.

Stop munching at night. This is by far the most difficult task, and it is where you will expend the majority of your energy. But remembered what David Sinclair said about hunger being a reminder of the good you're giving to your body during the day. As a result, condition your mind to accept those minor hunger pangs throughout the day. You know I will be able to eat shortly, and you are doing your part to improve your general health.

Use Himalayan rock salt to deceive your body into thinking it wasn't hungry. When you are hungry, put a few grains under your tongue and forget that you are hungry. You must be thinking if it would work, but it does!

I read that when you're fasting, you shouldn't take any vitamins because your body needs to perform all the job on its own. So that's what you should do.

When you break your fast, the first thing you should eat is protein. It has nothing to do with fat or carbohydrates. That will have a positive effect on your physique.

If you are having a really hectic day, perform a 20/4 fast so that you don't have to worry about food, meal preparation, or planning, depending on what you are doing.

Chapter 5: Kinds of Intermittent Fasting That Work Best for Women

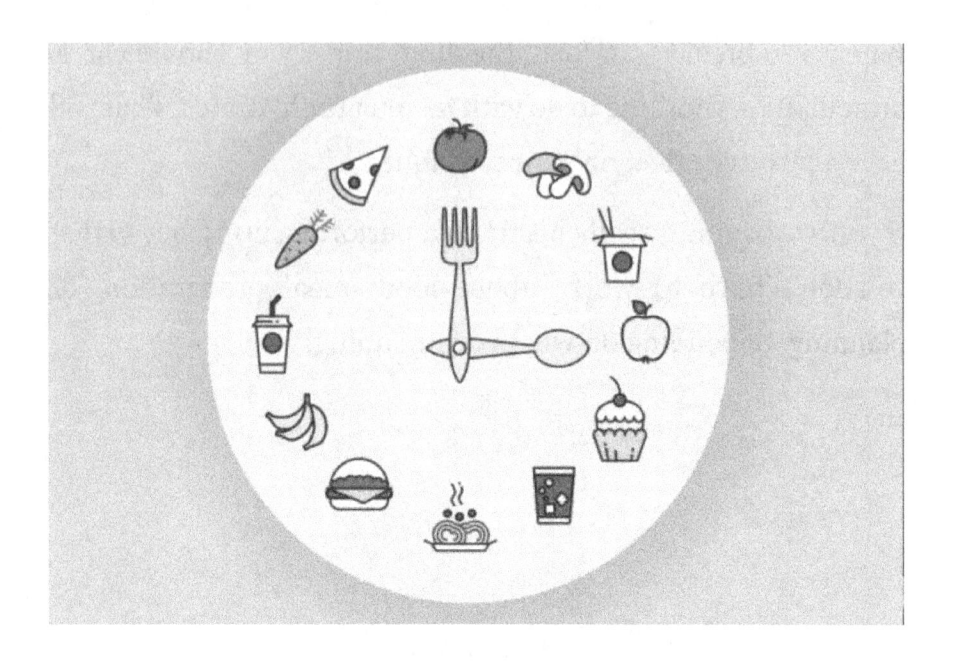

There is no such thing as a one-size-fits-all strategy to dieting. This holds true for intermittent fasting as well.

Women should, on average, adopt a more relaxed attitude to fasting than males.

Shorter fasting times, fewer fasting days, and/or taking a lower amount of calories on fasting days are all possible options.

Here are a some of the top intermittent fasting options recommended for women:

1. Method of Crescendo: Fasting for 12–16 hours twice or three times a week. Fasting days should not be consecutive and

should be spread out evenly during the week (for instance, Monday, Wednesday & Friday).

2. Eat-stop-& eat (also known as the 24-hour of protocol) is a dietary strategy in which you eat for a certain amount of time and then stop Once or also twice a week, go on a full 24-hour fast (max of two times a week for women). Begin with 14–16 hour fasts & work your way up.

3. The 5:2 Diet (also referred as "The Fast Diet") includes restricting calories to 25% of your regular intake (approximately 500 calories) for 2 days a week & eating "normal" for remaining five days. Fasting days should be separated by one day.

4. Fasting every day but eating normally on non-fasting days is known as modified alternate-day fasting. On a fasting day, you can ingest 20–25 percent of your normal calorie consumption (about 500 calories).

5. The 16/8 Approach (also known as the "Leangains method") entails fasting for 16 hours and eating all of your calories within about an eight-hour window. Women should start with 14-hour fasts & work their way up to 16 hours.

It is still crucial to eat well throughout the non-fasting periods, regardless of which option you choose. You may not see the same weight loss & health benefits if you eat many bad, calorie-dense items during the non-fasting periods.

At the end of your day, the optimal method is one that you can endure and maintain over time while not causing any detrimental health effects.

Chapter 6: Foods Women Over 50 Eat Should Eat in Intermittent Fasting

Please consult a health expert before making any big dietary changes to ensure that it is the smartest choice for you.

Intermittent fasting (IF) generates quite a stir in the congested world of dieting, despite the word "fasting" being very foreboding.

A fair amount of research (although with small sample sizes) shows that the diet can help women lose weight and control their blood sugar levels.

A reliable source It's no surprise that everybody and their aunt has jumped on the IF bandwagon.

Perhaps the attractiveness stems from the absence of food restrictions: you can eat when you want, but not necessarily what you want.

However, it's equally necessary to consider what's at stake. Should you be breaking your fast with pints of ice cream & bags of chips? Most likely not. That's why we've compiled a list of the greatest things to eat on an IF diet.

What should you actually eat when on IF?

Lauren Harris-Pincus, MS, RDN, writer of The Protein-Packed Breakfast Club, adds, "There are no stipulations or constraints concerning which type or how much food to eat while practicing intermittent fasting."

However, Mary Purdy, MS, RDN, chairman of Dietitians in Integrative & Functional Medicine, disagrees that "the advantages [of IF] are unlikely to accompany consistent Big Mac meals."

According to Pincus and Purdy, a well-balanced diet is a key to weight loss, maintaining energy levels, & sticking to the plan.

"Anyone trying to reduce weight should eat nutrient-dense foods including fruits, vegetables, whole grains, dairy, nuts, beans, seeds, and lean proteins," Pincus recommends.

"My recommendations would be quite similar to the meals I would generally recommend for optimal health — high-fiber, unprocessed, whole foods which offer variety & flavor," Purdy says.

To put it another way, if you eat many of the things listed below, you won't be hungry while fasting.

6.1 Water

OK, so this isn't strictly food, but it's incredibly vital for surviving IF.

Water is essential for the health of almost all of your body's major organs. Avoiding this as parts of your fast would be unwise. Your organs play a critical role in keeping you alive.

The volume of water that each individual should drink depends on their gender, height, weight, degree of exercise, and climate.

A reliable source, However, the color of your urine is a good indicator. At all times, you like it to be pale yellow.

Dehydration, which can induce headaches, weariness, and lightheadedness, is indicated by dark yellow urine. When you combine it with a lack of food, you have a recipe for failure — or, at the very minimum, pretty dark pee.

If plain water doesn't appeal to you, try adding a squeeze of lemon juice, several mint leaves, or cucumber slices to it.

Here's why H2O reigns supreme.

6.2 Avocado

Eating the highest-calorie fruit when attempting to reduce weight may seem paradoxical. But, on the other hand, avocados will keep you full throughout even the most stringent fasting times due to higher unsaturated fat content.

Unsaturated fats, according to research, keep the body full even though you don't feel hungry.

A reliable source Your body sends out signals that it doesn't need to go into urgent hunger mode since it has adequate nourishment. Even if you're hungry in the midst of a fasting period, unsaturated fats maintain these indications are continuing for longer.

Another study discovered that including half an avocado in your lunch would help you stay full for hours extra than if you don't eat the green, mushy fruit.

6.3 Seafood and fish

There's a reason why the American Dietary Guidelines recommend 2 to 3 four-ounce portions of fish per week.

In contrast to being high in healthy fats & protein, Trusted Source is also high in vitamin D.

And if you prefer to eat during restricted window times, don't you want to get an extra nutritional bang for your buck when you are doing it?

You'll never run out of the ways to prepare fish because there are so many options.

6.4 Cruciferous vegetables

The f-word – fiber — is abundant in foods like Brussels sprouts, broccoli, and cauliflower.

It's critical to eat fiber-rich foods regularly to keep you regular and ensure that your poop factory runs efficiently.

Fiber could also make you feel full, which is beneficial if you won't eat for another 16 hours.

Cruciferous vegetables can also help you avoid cancer.

6.5 Potatoes

Repeat after us: White foods aren't all awful.

In the 1990s, the researchers discovered that potatoes were one of the most satiating foods.

a reliable source, a 2012 study recognized that including potatoes in a healthy diet can aid in weight loss. (Sorry, but potato chips and French fries don't count.)

6.6 Legumes and beans

On the IF diet, your favorite chili topping could be your best friend.

Food, primarily carbohydrates, provides energy for physical activity. We're not suggesting you go crazy with carbs, but including low-calorie carbs like beans & legumes in your diet can't hurt. This can help you stay awake during your fasting period.

Furthermore, meals like chickpeas, peas, black beans, & lentils have been demonstrated to help people lose weight even when they aren't on a diet.

6.7 Probiotics

What do the little critters in the gut prefer to eat the most? Both consistency and variety are important. When they're hungry, this suggests they're not pleased. And if your gut isn't happy, you might notice some unpleasant side effects, such as constipation.

Add probiotic-rich foods to your diets, such as kefir, kombucha, and sauerkraut, to combat this discomfort.

6.8 Berry

These smoothie essentials are packed with vitamins and minerals. But that's not even the most exciting aspect.

Persons who ate a lot of flavonoids, such as those found in blueberries & strawberries, had lower BMI rises over 14 years than individuals who didn't eat berries, according to a 2016 study.

6.9 Eggs

One big egg has 6.24 grams of protein and takes only minutes to cook. And, especially when you're eating less, obtaining the same or more protein as possible is critical for staying full and growing muscle.

Those who ate an egg breakfast rather than a bagel were less hungry & ate less during the day, according to a 2010 study.

To put it another way, if you're searching for something to do throughout your fast, why not hard-boil a bunch of eggs? Then, when the moment is appropriate, you can eat them.

6.10 Nuts and seeds

Although nuts are heavier in calories than most snacks, they do include something that other snacks do not: healthy fats.

Also, don't be concerned about calories! According to a 2012 study, a 1-ounce serving of almonds (around 23 nuts) contains 20% fewer calories than the label claims. a reliable source

Chewing does not entirely break down the cell walls of almonds, according to the study. This keeps a nut section intact and prevents it from being absorbed by your body during digestion. As a result, eating almonds may not make as much of a difference in your daily calories as you may think.

6.11 Consume whole grains

Dieting and carbohydrate consumption seem to belong in 2 different categories. This isn't always the case, as you'll be relieved to learn. Because whole grains are high in fiber and protein, a small amount will keep you satisfied for a long time. a reliable source

So get out of your comfort zone and try farro, bulgur, spelt, Kamut, sorghum, amaranth, millet, or freekeh, a whole-grain nirvana.

Chapter 7: Foods Women Over 50 Should Avoid

7.1 Sugar

Sugar that has been refined serves to boost insulin levels in the body, which promotes fat storage. Unfortunately, it also affects the immune system, making it more difficult to fight infections and infections. So, the very next time you go for an additional slice of cake, consider your waistline.

7.2 Aerated beverages

Aerated drinks include empty calories that contribute to weight gain, not to mention the high sugar content. Fructose and other chemicals are used to make this sugar. This type of sugar is difficult to burn off, particularly around the midsection. Artificial sweeteners are also used in diet drinks, which are harmful to one's health.

7.3 Products derived from milk

Lactose intolerance, which can be minor or severe, is generally accompanied by gas. Reduce your intake of cheese, yogurt, & ice cream if you're feeling bloated. Choose lactose-free milk if you detect a difference.

7.4 Meat

If you can't eliminate meat from your diet, cutting back on it is a quick method to lose weight.

7.5 Alcohol

Because alcohol depresses the central nervous system, it decreases your metabolism. When alcohol is introduced to an elevated, high-calorie meal, a British study discovered that less adipose carbohydrate was burnt and more were retained as body fat. As a result, rather than a glass of red wine, it's advisable to wash down the meals with water.

7.6 Carbohydrates

Refined carbs, such as bread, potatoes, and rice, cause an insulin spike, lowering your basal metabolic rate. Additionally, when people reduce their carb intake, their appetite decreases and their weight loss.

7.7 Foods that have been fried

Although French fries could be your snack mix, they are oily and low in vitamins, minerals, and fiber. On the other hand, Fried foods are high in sodium and trans-fat, both of which cause stomach discomfort.

7.8 Salt in excess

Sodium, commonly found in packaged foods due to the ability to retain and enhance flavor, is one of the leading causes of a rounded stomach. It increases water retention and, therefore, can induce stomach bloating. In addition, when ingested in excess, sodium can cause severe changes in blood pressure.

Chapter 8: Weekly Meal Plan for Women Over 50

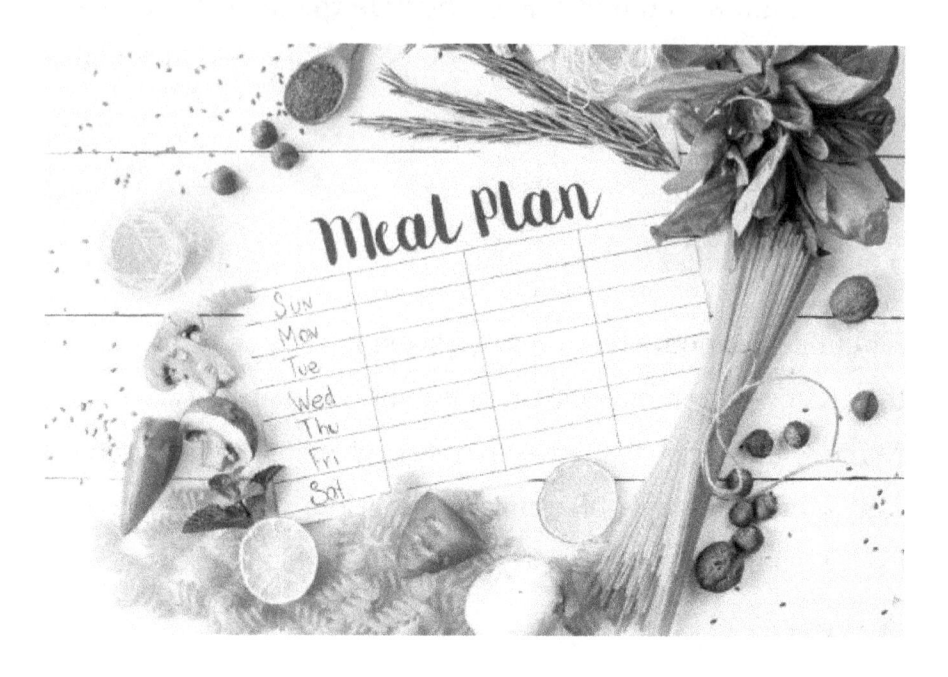

Before we get started on the intermittent fasting food plan, it's vital to grasp the difference between intermittent fasting and normal fasting. While there are several approaches to this, most individuals use the 16/8 technique, which entails eating for 8 hours & fasting for other 16 hours. There are, however, a variety of techniques that people might use. The goal is for a person to go without eating for a while, and when they do eat, they should avoid processed foods & focus on whole-food dishes.

Although many individuals prefer to forgo breakfast or supper, the technique does not force you to do so. You should also be aware that your calorie intake may vary depending on your body's weight-loss requirements. In general, meals which lean meats, include fish, healthy grains, and lots of vegetables, should be prioritized. The idea is that you'll eat a few larger meals, yet your total calorie intake will be lower because you'll only be eating within a specific window.

Day 1

1. For Breakfast: Baked Eggs with Spinach and Parmesan
2. For Lunch: Crispy Fish Tacos from the Oven
3. For Dinner: Skillet Turkey Burritos for Dinner
4. For the Snack: Dark Chocolate as a Snack (suggested two squares)

Day 2

1. For Breakfast: Breakfast Bowl with Hummus
2. For Lunch: Foil Pack of Baked Lemon Salmon & Asparagus
3. For Dinner: Stir-fried chicken and broccoli
4. For Snack: Boiled egg as a snack

Day 3

1. For Breakfast: Protein Pancakes with 4 Ingredients
2. For Lunch: Moroccan Couscous with Wild Cod
3. For Dinner: Stir-fried Honey and Garlic Shrimp
4. For Snack: Almonds as a snack (suggested 12-14)

Day 4

1. For Breakfast: Breakfast Cups with Ham and Eggs
2. For Lunch: Skillet with Sweet Potatoes and Turkey
3. For Dinner: Lemon Flavored White Fish Fillets
4. For Snack: 2 celery stalks with peanut butter

Day 5

1. For Breakfast: Oatmeal and Raisin Energy Bites No-Baked
2. For Lunch: Quinoa Cucumber Salad with Ground Turkey, Feta, and Olives
3. For Dinner: Skinny Salmon, Cashew, and Kale Bowl
4. For Snack: 1 cup of fresh strawberries as a snack

Day 6

1. For Breakfast: Green Creamy Smoothie with a Touch of Mint
2. For Lunch: Spring Rolls with Baked Chicken and Vegetables
3. For Dinner: Meatloaf of Skinny Turkey
4. For Snack: Avocado with tomatoes

Day 7

1. For Breakfast: Hash of Sweet Potatoes
2. For Lunch: Salad with Spicy Black Beans and Shrimp
3. For Dinner: Peppered Turkey Sausage with Onions
4. For Snack: 2 cups celery and carrots, chopped

Are you ready to give an intermittent fasting meal plan a try? Keep in mind that the specifics of your diet will vary depending on just how much calories you need to lose weight. In addition, for a meal plan to be far more successful, you'll need to determine your needed calorie intake.

Chapter 9: Frequently Asked Questions

Is it possible to work out when fasting?

Working exercise with IF may enhance the health advantages of both regimes, according to research. Participants who maintained an exercise regimen lost more weight than those who simply exercised or fasted in a 12-week research utilizing the 5:2 protocol (5 days of regular eating, followed by 2 days of reduced calories).

Some IF experts advise fasting overnight & exercising first thing in the morning. Glycogen reserves in your muscles are reduced after fasting overnight. As a result, your body will burn more fat to power your workout.

When I'm not fasting, what should I eat?

The majority of IF studies do not give specific recommendations for what to consume throughout your feeding window. However, whatever of the sort of fasting you select, make sure you're getting enough good calories throughout your feeding window. Avoid sugar and processed carbohydrates in favor of nutritious meals, including healthy fats, fiber-rich carbs, and protein (about 12-18 ounces per day).

Because some of the benefits of fasting come from lowering insulin production, it's become fashionable to combine it with a low-carb or keto diet. While you're not fasting, we encourage eating high-quality foods.

When it comes to intermittent fasting, how long would it take to become acclimated to it?

According to Krista Varady, a nutrition expert and fasting researcher, your body might want at least five days to acclimatize to the new eating and fasting routine.

To make the change simpler, experts recommend that newbies start with wider eating windows and progressively increase fasting time periods. They claim that feeling a bit hungry is beneficial because it promotes a stronger mind-body connection.

Is Intermittent Fasting safe for me?

Moderate fasting is beneficial to the majority of people (shorter than 24 hours). However, there are worries about the safety of pregnant women, children, people with type 1 diabetes, and those who are underweight or are not getting enough nourishment. Intermittent fasting is not recommended for these people, and they should see their doctor before doing this in the future.

Is it true that intermittent fasting can help you live longer?

Animal studies have shown that dietary restriction, such as caloric restriction & intermittent fasting, can prolong healthy longevity and postpone disease aging in a variety of species ranging from yeast to mice and to monkeys. The removal or enhanced functioning of senescent cells, or destroy cells which have been recognized by the body and prohibited from proliferating, is one of the molecular mechanisms underlying these effects. Intermittent fasting may prepare senescent cells for the cellular recycling, which may help aged tissues function better.

However, studying aging & senescence cell biomarkers in humans is difficult, especially because most people are unable or unwilling to engage in long-term intervention research. Human data from such research are uncommon, and the disciplines of calorie restriction and intermittent fasting are no exception.

While intermittent fasting (IF) has the potential to enhance tissue function, especially in terms of metabolic function & circadian rhythms, additional study on the effects of long-term fasting on the health span & longevity is needed.

Will I still need to count calories while fasting to lose weight?

Many people achieve natural caloric restriction & weight reduction without counting calories when they follow a time-restricted eating plan (such as a 16:8 fasting pattern). Dr. Krista Varady discovered that after three months of time-restricted feeding, most research participants automatically lowered their calorie intake by 300 calories on average and dropped 3% of their body weight, despite being told to eat regularly.

How can intermittent fasting help to slow down the aging process?

Intermittent fasting, according to researchers, can help people fight obesity, diabetes, & heart disease, all of which are major risk factors for age-related disorders like Alzheimer's.

According to animal research, intermittent dietary restriction reduces brain inflammation and preserves nerve cells. Autophagy, a cellular process in which the body breaks down & recycles worn-out cell components, is also activated.

IF encourages the production of growth hormone of human, that aids in the preservation of lean muscle mass & increases fat burning.

When I'm fasting, how do I deal with brain fog or fatigue?

Drink lots of water each day, whether you're fasting or not. According to some dietitians, calorie-free black coffee might assist with energy and focus. Meditation and other mindfulness practices may also assist with brain fog.

Low-impact exercise or moderate physical activity are good options. With IF, some people report having more energy and lucidity.

Should I continue to fast even if I am near to my ideal weight?

Enhanced insulin sensitivity, fat oxidation, and decreased inflammation are all possible advantages of intermittent fasting that are not related to weight reduction. Even if you don't like to lose weight, you can still adopt IF; however, you will need to make a deliberate effort to eat so much on your "feast" days or throughout your daily eating window to keep your present weight and energy consumption.

Dr. Krista Varady adds that those who don't want to lose weight might add some few calories to their fast days. She discovered that healthy persons lost 1/2 a pound per week on average when practicing alternate day fasting, but obese people lost 2-3 pounds per week. "Healthy people should make sure they consume enough calories and keep track of their weight to avoid falling into the underweight group. However, even if individuals lose only a small amount of weight, they can expect to experience metabolic benefits."

Conclusion

Even if you are only adjusting when you eat items, it is always best to talk with a certified healthcare practitioner before making dietary adjustments. They can help you figure out if intermittent fasting is right for you. This is especially crucial for longer-term fasts that may result in vitamin and mineral deficiency. It's critical to recognize that your bodies are quite sophisticated. If food is limited at one meal, the body may experience increased appetite and calorie consumption at the following meal, as well as a slowing of metabolism to match caloric intake. Although intermittent fasting has some possible health benefits, this should not be believed that if rigorously followed, it will result in massive weight loss & prevent the onset of disease progression. It's a valuable tool, but a combination of tools may be required to achieve and sustain optimal health.